Essential Oils:
Detox Your Environment

A. L. Elder

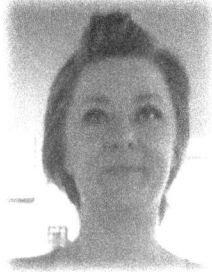

Hi! My name is April, and I am thrilled you decided to purchase a copy of my Essential Oil: Detox Your Environment, book! I am so excited to share with you all of the many things we have done with our essential oils to clean up around our home. Truth be told, I have taken a lot of these recipes to the office and I use them there as well!

When I began researching essential oils, I discovered a company and fell in love with their mission statement. I ordered my first batch of oils and lined them up on my desk. I wasn't really too sure what I expected, I just wanted to incorporate them into our lives. Oh! I'm sorry, I forgot we were doing the introduction and here I am rushing along about the oils!

I am married to a wonderful guy whose patience has been tested time and time again…not intentionally by me of course! But, any of you who are married can understand, we girls' can get our minds set to something and there's not a darn thing our husbands can do to change those plans! He was pretty skeptical about incorporating essential oils into our daily lives. That was, until we made the laundry detergent recipe you will find in this book. We made five gallons of laundry detergent for less than five dollars. Of course, he came around pretty quickly after that!

I work full time, I write books, and I am one the most unorganized person you have ever met when it comes to recipe cards…seriously, before writing this book, my desk was cluttered with 3 x 5 cards!

In 2012, I began researching ways to improve our overall health. Oh geeze, I was not your poster child of wellness! I was over-weight, addicted to sugar and processed everything. I began writing a comical memoir about my weight and discovered something truly amazing. I had the choice to continue being unhealthy, or I had the choice to make significant changes to become healthy once again. While the idea began with eating whole foods and detoxing from sugar, caffeine, high-fructose corn syrup—it really evolved into something more when I discovered essential oils.

I quickly turned our kitchen into an essential oils lab. I concocted everything from chap stick to laundry detergent in a matter of weeks. I was on a mission to rid our environment of everything toxic. This is when I decided to write this book. I had successfully integrated essential oils into cleaning and detoxing the air we breathe inside our home and wanted to share my recipes with everyone wanting to incorporate them too. I also wanted to create a place where I could organize them and find them all in one place. Before writing this book, I had recipes scattered from one end to another on my desk at home. I rated all of the recipes I came across and finally chose our favorites to publish for you.

I chose to incorporate therapeutic grade essential oils. I purchase mine at wholesale, direct from the company, and I know the oils I receive are 100% pure. I don't have to worry about the oils staining my clothes, furniture, or wonder if they contain fillers like alcohol. They are super potent, so less is really more.

If you want to know more about the brand of oils I use, please feel free to email me at a.l.elder2012@gmail.com and I will share them with you. If you have already made your choice, wonderful! If, though, your oils are not 100% pure, your results may vary from mine.

Since this book is to share uses, I did use the generic name of all the oil blends. If you are not sure which blend coincides with the blend I have listed feel free to email me, and I will do my best to research the different blends and let you know.

Contents

Crazy Lady

"You use them for what?"

This is the common reaction I receive when I share my uses for essential oils. I know, I know…I should wear a flower in my hair and smell like patchouli…then perhaps people would take me seriously. The truth is, I love my oils and I am not some crazy lady pushing snake oils or magic potions! How many of you have had a similar reaction from your friends and family? Don't worry, we are not all crazy! In fact, I haven't met a single oil user who I identified as crazy at all. We are all simply looking for ways to clean up and incorporate natural products rather than filling our homes and bodies with chemicals.

So, should we get started on some recipes?

The Bathroom

The bathroom contains so many places where germs and bacteria thrive! Even the occasional spores of mold have been located on the shower curtain liner in our home. (Gross and dangerous!) So, here are my tried and true recipes for cleaning the bathroom without having to open all the windows and doors because with these recipes…there are absolutely no toxins! You can breathe easy and my recipes contain oils which can lift your mood! (I know, just a little bonus for those of us who dread cleaning the bathroom!)

Tub, tile and sinks:

1 Glass Bowl
1 cup Baking Soda
½ cup Borax
2 drops Melaleuca Oil
5 drops Lemon Oil
1 Glass Parmesan Cheese Shaker*
1 Funnel

Mix/mash all ingredients in a glass bowl until well combined. Using your funnel, transfer the mixed powder to the parmesan shaker. (The kind you see in pizza parlors.) Sprinkle in you toilet bowl, tub, shower and sinks. Wet a sponge or cleaning cloth to scrub the areas. Rinse and enjoy the shine as well as the fresh smell!

Melaleuca oil is anti-fungal, anti-bacterial and anti-microbial! In a nut shell: if there was something growing in those areas, more than likely you have taken care of the problem!

Lemon oil is a mood lifter. The bright aroma fills your senses with happiness, and let's just admit once and for all…not many of us enjoy being on our hands and knees in front of the commode!

Lemon is also antioxidants and recommended for cleaning and purifying. (Again, I love that it brightens my mood while I am cleaning. It is not my favorite thing to do!)

*You may also use a canning jar! Simply poke holes in the lid as you did when you were a kid to keep grasshoppers and fireflies.

To store: Place a piece of plastic wrap between the lid and glass. Then tighten down. This will help keep moisture from locking your cleaner into a hard white pumice stone.

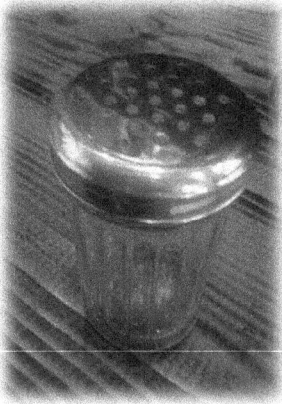

Parmesan Cheese Shaker

Extra Scrubbing Power

1 cup Baking Soda
½ cup Borax
¼ cup Water
2 drops Melaleuca Oil
5 drops Orange Oil

Mix/mash all ingredients in a glass bowl until well combined. Add water to make a paste for extra scrubbing power. This works well for grout and water stains!

Melaleuca is also referred to as Tea Tree Oil. It has a wonderful, clean and crisp scent of earthy-rosemary and pine. A perfect choice for its anti-fungal properties!

Orange Oil, for me, is a soothing smell. While it is a bright and super clean fragrance, it reminds me of my childhood. My mom would put orange rinds and cinnamon sticks in a cast iron tea pot atop the woodstove in our living room. The orange peel would release the oils and our home always smelled amazing during the winter months.

Counters and floors:

I personally recommend glass spray bottles for all of your cleaners. They are super easy to find with a quick Internet search. Mine are cobalt blue, but you can choose any color you want. I use an eight-ounce bottle. I recommend having six on hand, although you could probably get away with only four. I mix my cleaners each time I plan on cleaning the house. So, for me, it's every week. (I do have a counter cleaner ready at all times, though. That one is used multiple times a day. I also made one for my office at work!)

Counter Cleaner:

6 drops Orange oil
4 drops Melaleuca oil
3 drops Lemon oil
Water
1 8 oz. Glass Spray Bottle

Add oils to your glass bottle. Fill with water and shake well. Spray on counters and faucets the wipe with a dry cloth. (Yes, that's it!)

It works amazingly fast to break down and make-up or toothpaste adhered to the bathroom counters! And the aroma!!! Talk about going to a happy place!! I love combining the citrus oils with the Melaleuca. Fresh, clean and non-toxic!

Floor Cleaner:

1/4 c Hot Water
1/4 c White Distilled Vinegar
1/4 c 70% Isopropyl (Rubbing) Alcohol
2 drops Melaleuca oil (anti-bacterial and anti-fungal)
1 drop Purifying Blend oil (Sanitizer)
1 drop Protective Blend oil (good for everything!!)
1 drop of liquid dish detergent
1 8 oz. Glass Spray Bottle

I use an 8 oz. glass bottle with a sprayer and simply mix the ingredients in a glass measuring cup. Use a funnel to transfer from the measuring cup to the bottle.

Spray a very fine mist over and area (2'x5'-ish) and let set for a couple of seconds to allow the solution an opportunity to break down the dirt. I use a microfiber mop...I have to rinse the microfiber often due to my muddy footed, four-legged friend.

Super quick drying time...no streaks and the house smells amazing!

8 oz. is what I use every weekend on our floors.

(1200-ish square feet) I simply mix up a new batch each time. The hot water helps to break down the heavy traffic areas.

Mirrors & Glass Cleaner

You are going to FLIP over this one! We tried a lot of different recipes before finally combining our favorites into one! This one takes the cake! No streaks, smells ahhh-mazing and does an amazing job on both mirrors and windows.

¼ cup Distilled White Vinegar
¼ cup 70% Isopropyl (Rubbing) Alcohol
1 T. Cornstarch
2 cups Hot Water (just from your tap)
4 drops Lavender oil (calms and relaxes)
2 drops Castile Liquid Soap
1 empty (plastic) glass cleaner bottle (I recycled the store-bought one)

Oh…and a funnel, unless you can mix it all in a large measuring cup with a pour spout.

Combine the vinegar, rubbing alcohol, Lavender and Castile liquid soap and set aside.

Combine the water and cornstarch in another bowl and whisk until combined/dissolved.

Using your funnel, combine all ingredients and VIOLA! I use old newspaper instead of paper towels to clean my mirrors and windows. Shake well between uses to ensure the cornstarch is still combined. Otherwise, it may plug up the sprayer.

Another tip: Use less! This is a super concentrated glass cleaner! Less is definitely more!

The Kitchen

Did you know studies have found more bacteria living in the kitchen sink than on the toilet seat of your commode? Okay, so if you haven't heard that already it sounds pretty gross, right? But, if you think about, we really do use our kitchen sinks to get rid of, rinse off and dispose of many things.

Wooden Cutting Boards

7 drops Lemon oil
30 drops Fractionated Coconut Oil

Use a dry dishcloth to rub the oil into your cutting board. Not only have you disinfected the board, you are helping preserve it for many, many years to come.

Fractionated Coconut Oil will not turn rancid. It is colorless and odorless as well. The Lemon Oil cleans and sanitizes the wood, plus it is all natural! You don't have to worry about toxic chemicals lingering and waiting for the fresh foods you will cut and eventually feed your family!

Stainless Steel Appliances

1 old/clean sock
20 drops Fractionated Coconut Oil
5 drops Orange Oil

Place the sock over your hand like a sock-puppet. Simply add the oils to the area where your fingers are. Clean your appliances with circular motions and then stand back and admire the shine!

Our appliances never looked so good! Okay, maybe when they were first installed, but this little recipe is amazing. I love how the kitchen smells of oranges too! So fresh, so clean and all natural!

I usually only need to clean ours every other week! The oils help prevent fingerprints!

Glass Stovetop Cleaner

1/3 cup Baking Soda
5 drops Melaleuca Oil
3 clean dish towels
Hot water

Combine the baking soda and Melaleuca in a glass bowl. Sprinkle lightly over your glass cooktop.

Take the three clean dishtowels and wet each of them in the hottest water you can stand. Ring them out until damp and place over the cooktop.

Let sit for ten minutes and then use the dishtowels to remove the baking soda mixture. Dry your cooktop and enjoy the shine!

When rinsing your dishtowels, you can also use the residual cleaning solution to scrub your sink! This one is a two-for-one!

Counter Tops

6 drops Orange oil
4 drops Melaleuca oil
3 drops Protective Blend oil
1 8 oz. Glass Spray Bottle

Add the oils to your glass bottle and fill with water. Shake well between uses. Spray directly onto counter tops and clean with a sponge or dish cloth.

Laminate Floor Cleaner

See the same recipe under bathroom floor cleaner.

Coffee Pot Cleaner (Drip)

6 cups Distilled White Vinegar
4 cups Water
8 drops Lime Oil
2 drops Lemon Oil

Combine all ingredients in the carafe and pour into reserve. Run one cycle with cleaning solution and three cycles with just water.

All of the ingredients are natural and aid in breaking down hard water and mineral build-up in your coffee maker.

The oils will not leave a residue and I promise…your coffee will not taste "citrusy"…it will simply taste like coffee!

Dishwasher Detergent (Powder)

2 cups Borax
2 cups Washing Soda
1 cup Epsom Salt
10 packages Unsweetened Lemonade (citric acid)
15 drops Lavender Oil*
An air-tight container to store it in

Mix all ingredients in a bowl and place in an air-tight container. (Oh my word...this one is so quick and easy!)

I use a 1/4 measuring cup, but only fill it 1/2 way with the detergent.

SUPER DUPER EASY!!

*You can substitute Lime, Lemon or Orange Oils too!

Laundry Day

My very least favorite responsibility of being an adult has got to be doing laundry! Seriously, there are only two of us and I swear we produce far too many "dirty" clothes! I used to purchase laundry detergent at the store. I used to use fabric softener and dryer sheets too. That was before I discovered they all contain cancer-causing toxins! Yes, ladies and gents…cancer-causing chemicals. Now, I don't know about you, but this discovery actually frightened me!

I knew I had options and I made three different batches of laundry detergent before choosing this recipe to share with you. Now, I have a septic system, so I was really careful about what I was putting down our drain. There is some controversy about using Borax, (totally Internet search if you are curious,) but for us…this was our solution. There are absolutely no cancer-causing agents in this recipe!

Liquid Laundry Detergent (Liquid)

1 Five Gallon Bucket with an airtight lid
1 Bar of Soap
2 qt. Water
2 cups Borax
1 cup Baking Soda
2 cups Washing Soda
50 drops Lemongrass Oil (you can substitute
Lavender too)

Put 2 quarts of water in a large saucepan and
turn it on low. Grate the bar soap. (I used a very
fine grater.) Put the grated soap in the saucepan
and stir constantly until melted and combined.
Remove from heat and set aside. (TIP: Please do
this step slowly. If your water begins to boil, you
will have suds from one end of your kitchen to the
other.)

Place the Borax, baking soda and Washing
Soda into the five-gallon bucket and add four and a
half gallons of very hot tap water. Stir to combine.
Add the bar soap/water mixture and stir once
more. Place lid on bucket and store at room
temperature for 24-48 hours. Stir once more and
then you are ready to use it!

I recycle my old laundry detergent container. I use a funnel and glass mixing cup to transfer the detergent to the container. For a little extra fabulousness, I add twenty drops of Lemongrass oil to the detergent each time I refill.

Dryer Balls

Remember what I wrote about dryer sheets? While, yes, they make your clothes smell amazing and feel so soft: is it really worth it? I found a wonderful alternative to dryer sheets! They are 100% pure and natural. The best part is, we use them over and over and over again!

Before we get to those…do you have static cling issues? Us too!! Okay, so now that we ditched the dryer sheets, we use aluminum foil for static cling! Just tear off a sheet about the size you would to cover a casserole dish and crumple it into a ball. Toss it into the dry and boom! No more static cling!

Is that not too cool? I am always amazed when I find something so easy!

Wool-Felted Dryer Balls

2 skeins Wool Yarn (Any color...your choice)
1 pair old nylons (knee highs work perfectly!)
1 large Yarn Needle

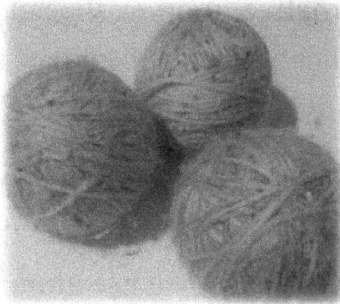

Oh my goodness! This is so super easy! So, all you need to do is roll your wool yarn into balls about the size of tennis balls. Once completed: cut the yarn leaving about two inches. Thread your yarn needle and bring the needle and the "tail" straight through the middle of your dryer ball. I recommend making 6-8 dryer balls at a time. Now, place one ball at a time into the leg of one nylon, tying a very tight knot in between each ball. Place the caterpillar-looing string in the washing machine and wash on HOT. Then, toss them into the dryer (still in the nylon) and dry them completely. (It's fine if you throw your laundry in with them.) Once completely dried/felted, remove them from the nylons.

You will need to repeat the nylon/washing/drying process about every 600 load of laundry. You will know when because the yarn begins to pull away from the ball.

We use the balls (4 balls) in every load of laundry we put into the dryer. I love them! They soften our clothes and actually shorten the drying time, so we are conserving energy too!

Here are some of our favorite oils to add to our dryer balls:

> Lavender (bedding)
> Lavender and Lemongrass (towels)
> Melaleuca and Orange (sneakers)
> Cedar Wood (lap quilts and blankets)

Add two drops of your favorite oil(s) to each dryer ball. We do about eight loads of laundry a week and we only add oils once: right before we throw our first load into the dryer.

I like having multiple dryer balls with different oils on them so I can mix-and-match as I am doing different items.

Breathe Easy

Let's talk about the air in your home. It should be the single place you and your family are breathing pure, unadulterated, chemical and toxin free air, right?

Now, you are talking to a girl who used to have a candle punch card, here. I had NO IDEA some candles contained not only LEAD (!!!) but other artificial chemicals to enhance the overall aroma.

I am not going to tell you all candles and wax warmers are bad. But...I want you to think about your oils. They are 100% pure. No artificial additives. No chemicals. No toxins.

If you are investing in overall health and well-being...I recommend investing in pure air too!

The wonderful thing I love about my diffuser -vs- a candle or wax warmer is I can change the scent in minutes and at very little cost. The average cost per drop of oil is 12 cents!!

Diffusers

There are so many oil diffusers on the market today! There isn't a brand that I prefer over another. In fact, we have four different diffusers in our home and I have another in my office! Just be sure your diffuser is designed to be used with essential oils.

If a blend is too strong for you, try reducing the recipe by half. I have been diffusing for about six months now, so my scent tolerance is pretty high.

Something Smells Fishy

You have prepared a wonderful meal and the kitchen smells…well not as wonderful! This diffuser recipe works great for removing all sorts of odors from the air. Fish, bacon, man-cave…you name it! This one will definitely purify and remove those nasty odors!

70 ml Water
1 drop Cilantro Oil
1 drop Lemon Oil
1 drop Peppermint Oil
1 drop Orange Oil

Improve Your Mood

You've had a looooong day! Your mind is exhausted and there are a hundred things you need to get done before heading to bed. This recipe will definitely help motivate you! This is also a great blend to diffuse while working out!

70 ml Water
1 drop Wintergreen Oil
1 drop Orange
1 drop Cedar Wood

Focus, Focus, Focus

This is one of my favorites to diffuse when I am doing taxes, paying bills or simply feel totally distracted by shiny objects!

70 ml Water
1 drop Grapefruit Oil
1 drop Orange Oil
1 drop Lemongrass Oil

Give Thanks

Perfect blend for fall! This one smells like a warm hug feels. I hope that makes sense! It is a cozy and welcoming blend.

70 ml Water
1 drop Cinnamon Oil
1 drop Orange Oil
1 drop Clove Oil
1 drop Ginger Oil

Holiday Wreath

This one is also perfect if you have an artificial tree and miss the fragrance of a fresh-cut pine! Not too strong, this blend is refreshing!

70 ml Water
2 drops Cypress Oil
1 drop Juniper Berry Oil
1 drop Cassia Oil
1 drop White Fir Oil

Cedar Chest

I love this woodsy-fragrance! It brings the outside indoors and smells so refreshing! A very warm and earthy smell!

70 ml Water
3 drops Cedar Wood Oil
3 drops White Fir Oil
1 drop Juniper Berry Oil

No More Snoring

We diffuse this blend in our bedroom and we both sleep soundly. Um…one of used to snore…but, I don't anymore!

70 ml Water
2 drops Eucalyptus Oil
1 drop Melaleuca Oil
1 drop Lemon Oil

No More Nightmares

Little ones swear by this blend! I have personally made this blend for friends and they have started incorporating oils even more!

70 ml Water
4 drops Lavender Oil
1 drop Roman Chamomile Oil

Girly Girl

Wonderful blend for a girls' party at the house! This is one of my favorites to diffuse in my home office while I am typing away.

70 ml Water
2 drops Patchouli Oil
1 drop Geranium Oil
2 drops Ylang Ylang

Creepy Crawlers and Mice

I am so fortunate to live with nature. Our home is nestled amongst cedar, pine and wild blackberry bushes. We have an apple orchard where deer come every night to feed. They also bring their babies and we watch them from the porch. Ahhhh, so peaceful!

That is, until our yellow Labrador catches sight of them and takes of running through the orchard like a rabid beast. He chases them while barking his head off and wagging his tail. I have always thought he was sending a mixed message! Don't worry, though, our dog is slightly overweight and while he does give it his all…those deer are agile and quick!

Any who…we have bugs and giant spiders and mice who truly love the inside of our country home as much as we do! I have some tried and true recipes to deter them from entering.

Mice and cupboards

When I discovered the tale-tale signs that mice had invaded my lazy-Susan's in the kitchen I was utterly disgusted! Needless to say, I didn't require a black light to see what they had left behind. I cleaned all of my baking sheets and other miscellaneous from the cabinets and mixed up my mouse-deterrent cleaning solution. Then I tried something that I was pretty sure wasn't going to work, but hey, it was totally worth a shot, right?

All I had to lose was some mice. Guess what? It worked! It worked amazingly! You have to try this if you have mice invading your space.

Mice Pre-Cleaner

1 8 oz. Glass Spray Bottle
15 drops Peppermint Oil
5 drops Cypress Oil
Water

Combine oils in your glass bottle then fill with water. Spray the interior of the cupboards down liberally and wait 5-10 minutes before wiping down with paper towels. (Vacuum out the area first if you notice there is "solid" mice remnants!)

The Peppermint oil is super fragrant! Holy smokes, is it ever. Just a warning…you may experience some eye watering if you get into the mist produced by spraying this cleaner. Peppermint is naturally antibacterial and an antiseptic.

The Cypress oil contains antiseptic, antibacterial astringent properties. Plus, it totally smells clean and woodsy. Perfect for cleaning your wood cabinets!

Okay, so now that you have the cabinets sanitized…let's move on to the next step. (This is the one I was really skeptic about.)

Peppermint Mice Balls

1 Cottonball
3 drops Peppermint Oil

Place three drops of Peppermint oil on a cotton ball. Place the cottonball in your cabinet. That's it!

Okay, so the name of this recipe was a tough one to come up with. I know...it's a little...um, a little inappropriate?!

However, this really does work. When I tried this the first time, I had my husband put mouse traps in the cabinet alongside the peppermint cottonballs to see if they would deter the pesky little monsters. In the six month time frame we didn't catch a single mouse. I also didn't find anymore "evidence" they were exploring my lazy-Susan!

I replace the cottonballs every six months. (Okay, not really, I replace them when I think about which is more like every year!) I do recommend you do better than I and replace yours every six months.

Ants, Spiders and Fruit Flies

Oh the joy of insects! We have had our fair share and have come up with a few solutions we totally recommend you try.

Ants (All sorts of shapes and sizes)

1 8 oz. Glass Spray Bottle
5 drops Cilantro Oil
5 drops Melaleuca Oil
5 drops Peppermint Oil
Water

Combine the oils and water in your glass spray bottle. Now, go where the ants are exiting and entering your home. (It is not hard. Most of the time, in our house, there is a constant "ant line" from one area to another.)

Spray the area with a fine mist of your solution. Let dry. Repeat daily for a week then as needed.

Cilantro oil was a total discovery for me. I had notice the ants did not like it in my garden and decided to incorporate it into this recipe. So far...ants be gone!

Spider Repellant

1 8 oz. Glass Spray Bottle
12 drops Peppermint Oil
8 drops Rosemary Oil
Water

Combine oils in your glass spray bottle and fill with water. Spritz around the baseboards inside your home. I also spray this is my garden!

Rosemary oil has long been used as a fumigant! (I know, right?) So, with this in mind, and know my other "peskies" didn't like Peppermint, I combined the two.

I much prefer the smell of Peppermint and Rosemary to the over-the-counter fumigation spray cans! And honestly, the bugs live…just not inside our home!

Fruit Flies Be Gone

1 Glass Bowl
¼ cup Apple Cider Vinegar
1 drop Blue Dish Detergent
1 drop Grapefruit Oil
1 T. Water

Combine all ingredients in a glass bowl. Place the bowl near where the fruit flies are active. Replace every 24 hours until the fabulous fruit flies are no longer invading your kitchen!

I added the Grapefruit oil because…well, they are fruit flies, right? I have tried the recipe with out and I will be honest with you: the addition of the Grapefruit oil does make a positive difference in the amount of time it takes to rid your kitchen of the tiny buzzards!

Buzzards! That word just makes me laugh! Anyway, the Grapefruit oil also helps mask the vinegar scent of this recipe. Let's be honest, vinegar is amazing, but to smell it as an air freshener…yeh, not so much.

That's a wrap!

Well, those are my tried and true recipes for using essential oils to detox your environment! Again, I want to say thank you for purchasing my book and I hope you found some really great recipes to use in your home.

I also hope you found a few giggles hidden amongst the pages as well.

If you have any questions, feel free to reach out to me. I am in love with my essential oils and would definitely not hesitate to share more information about them with you.

If you have a moment, please leave a review where you purchased this book. Reviews help future readers choose a book and your review could be the one they see! Help them discover the many benefits of detoxing their environment too!

I have added some blank recipe cards in the back of the paperback version to help you, keep all of your favorite cleaning recipes together!

Thanks again!!

Recipe Card for: _____

_____
_____
_____
_____
_____
_____
_____
_____

_____
_____
_____
_____
_____
_____
_____
_____
_____
_____
_____
_____

Recipe Card for: _____

_____

_____

_____

_____

_____

_____

_____

_____

_____

_____

_____

_____

_____

_____

_____

_____

_____

_____

_____

_____

_____

Recipe Card for: _____

_____

_____

_____

_____

_____

_____

_____

_____

_____

_____

_____

_____

_____

_____

_____

_____

_____

_____

_____

_____

Recipe Card for: _____

_____

_____

_____

_____

_____

_____

_____

_____

_____

_____

_____

_____

_____

_____

_____

_____

_____

_____

_____

_____

Recipe Card for: _____

_____

_____

_____

_____

_____

_____

_____

_____

_____

_____

_____

_____

_____

_____

_____

_____

_____

_____

_____

_____

_____

_____

_____

_____

Recipe Card for: _____

_____

_____

_____

_____

_____

_____

_____

_____

_____

_____

_____

_____

_____

_____

_____

_____

_____

_____

_____

Contact the Author

Find her on Facebook:
https://www.facebook.com/april.l.elder.7

Email her:
a.l.elder2012@gmail.com

Follow her on twitter:
https://twitter.com/ALElderAuthor

Need a light-hearted book to lift your spirits? Need a little giggle?

Check out A. L. Elder on Amazon!

<u>Hey Lady…are these your underwear?</u>

A book filled with mostly true stories from the life of, A. L. Elder. This book takes the reader on a journey through childhood adventures, tenacious-teenage-tasks and adulthood mishaps. A comical look back at the moments in life when lessons were learned and crying was not an option. April survived the interrogation process of her parents'--learned that gilding and a gelding were two different things--and became a stalker to win the heart of her future husband.

Somewhere along the way, her skirt got tucked into her tights and her dog ate her underwear.

Who's the Girl in the Fat Suit?

Her mother warned her! She told April that one day all of the sodas and candy bars would catch up to her. When it happened, and yes, it happened…April stood shell-shocked in front of the bathroom mirror staring at her larger than life reflection.

Blaming a happy marriage, genes and the curse of her mother, April set out on a journey to improve her self-image. She tried everything from red and green highlights in her hair to piercings and acrylic nails, but still found the fat suit to be all consuming.

Who's the Girl in the Fat Suit is a true story of one woman's journey from a size four to a size twelve-ish. April struggled with self-acceptance and finally found her answer to weight loss, but not without failing and falling numerous times. This memoir is written in a blog-like style complete with quick and easy to read chapters.

If you have ever stood in front of a full-length mirror and asked, "Really?" You may enjoy

April's latest release: Who's the Girl in the Fat
Suit.

Thank you again for purchasing this book! I sincerely hope you try some of the recipes and you love them as much as we do!

I wish you all of the health and happiness in the world.

Kindest regards,
April

www.ingramcontent.com/pod-product-compliance
Lightning Source LLC
Chambersburg PA
CBHW060634280326
41933CB00012B/2031